Want free goodies?
Email us at freebies@honeybadgercoloring.com

@honeybadgercoloring

Honey Badger Coloring

Shop our other books at
www.honeybadgercoloring.com

Wholesale distribution through Ingram Content Group
www.ingramcontent.com/publishers/distribution/wholesale

For questions and customer service, email us at
support@honeybadgercoloring.com

I am a nice PERSON, Just don't PUSH MY BITCH button.

Want free goodies?
Email us at freebies@honeybadgercoloring.com

@honeybadgercoloring

Honey Badger Coloring

Shop our other books at
www.honeybadgercoloring.com

Wholesale distribution through Ingram Content Group
www.ingramcontent.com/publishers/distribution/wholesale

For questions and customer service, email us at
support@honeybadgercoloring.com

Made in the USA
Las Vegas, NV
17 December 2023

82967099R00059